To
Maritza,

Practice with purpo

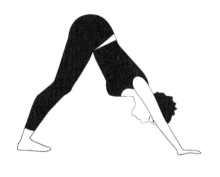

Om, the Poses You'll Do!

by
Lyn Gerfin

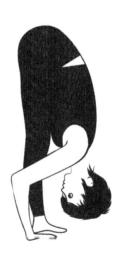

Illustrations by Katie Morgan

ISBN 978-0-692-06777-2

Editing: Carin L. Crook

IngramSpark Independent Publishing Platform
Printed in the USA

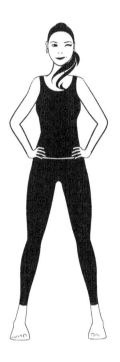

For My Students
Past, Present, and Future

Sun Salutations to you!
You've made up your mind.
You're off to start yoga!
Not sure what you'll find.

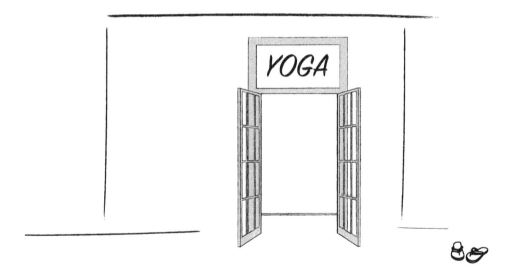

You have yoga pants on.
You have feet on your mat.
You can bend yourself forward,
and slightly bend back.

You feel somewhat nervous,
the teacher throws you a wink.
"Okay, not so bad.
I can do this," you think.

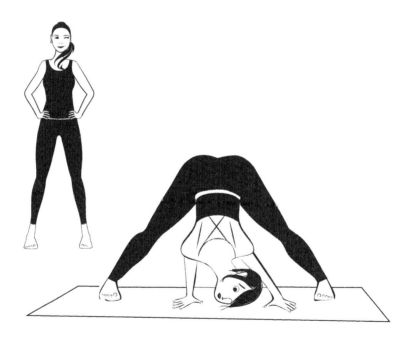

Now the temptation is there
to look left and look right.
Particularly at the student
in the hot pink yoga tights.

But stick with your Drishti,
your soft, steady gaze.
It will help you find clarity,
and get you out of your haze.

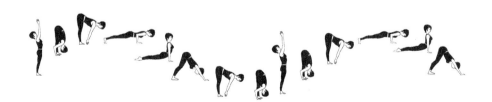

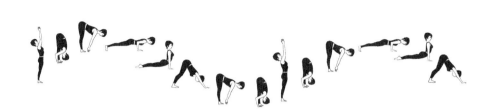

And you'll get mixed up a bit
when you first start to flow.
So just stay with the practice,
and see how it grows!

The teacher will say things
that at first seem confusing.
A lot of new words,
you may be consuming.

Ujjayi and Uddiyana,
yoga tools you are given.
Sukha and Sthira help find balance,
not make you driven.

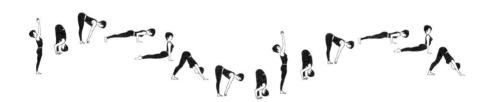

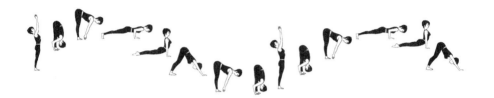

When that begins to happen,
resist the fight or the flight.
Have trust in the process,
you will find your inner light.

The understanding will come soon,
these words are really not scary.
Effort without tension,
and breathing, don't be wary.

There will be up dogs and flipped dogs,
a down dog or five.
Crows, instead of flying,
will choose to nose dive.

There will be twisting, backbending,
mountains to climb.
Some poses will feel as if
you're balancing on a dime.

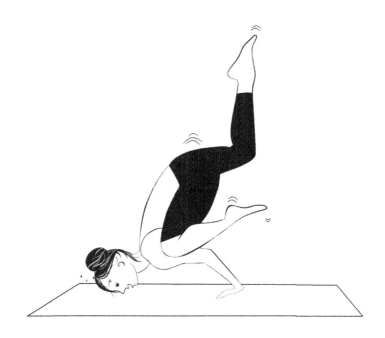

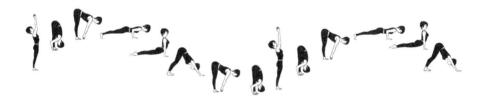

You will learn new maneuvers,
that are more than just awkward.
Tangle up your left and right,
stepping forward and backward.

And there will be a few poses
you really shouldn't do.
Your body will fight back,
your mind will muscle through.

You will huff, and you'll puff,
you will blow your pose down!

At this moment, my friend,
drop your knees to the ground.

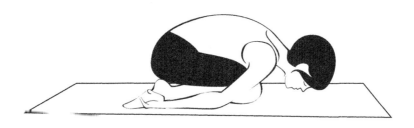

Take the Child's Pose view,
to rebuild your foundation.
There is power in a pause,
it's called transformation.

And then you will see,
it's not about bending.
In this case, it seems,
to be about breath never ending!

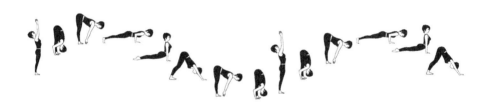

Somehow you'll move away
from doing and thinking.
You'll find that yoga zone
without even blinking.

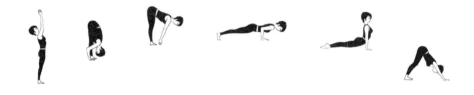

And oh, how you'll flow! You will, the flow grows!

With steadiness in breath,
and a release of frustration,
you will flow through the poses,
give yourself a silent ovation!

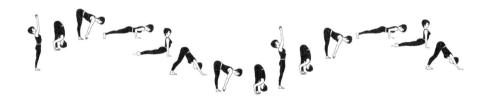

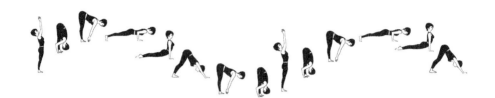

Om, the poses you'll do!
There are handstands to be done!
There are photos to take!
Airbrushing to some!

You will pose on the beach!
You will pose in the snow!
You will pose, sad to say,
places no pose should go.

You will be #instafamous!
A yogi rock star!
A *Yoga Journal* cover!
The dreams will go far!

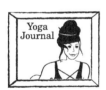 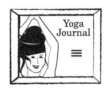 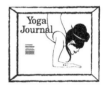

You will be the best yogi
of Instagram fame!

Until your mat slips out from under,
your ego goes down in flames...

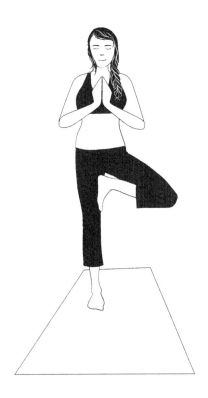

And back alone you will be,
just your mat and your Self.
That unbearable sound of stillness,
where you will find some great wealth.

You see…

You can't be bad at yoga,
and you also can't be good.
You can't do it with ego,
I can'ts, or I shoulds.

All you can do is the practice,
the process is the key.
Put the tools to work,
and you will find what you need.

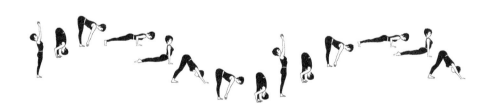

And it won't always be easy,
this yoga path way.
When times get a bit rough,
you might think "nah-amnotgonna-stè."

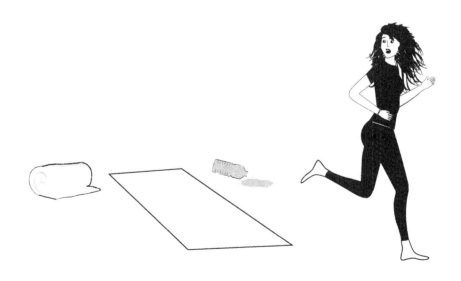

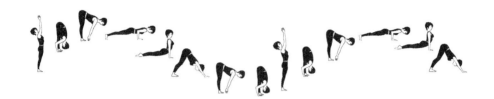

But practice you will
on days you feel blue.
Practice you will
when friends aren't true.

You see practice you'll find
is the *only* way through.

Practice on some days
might need a few tweaks.
Your toes might get sore,
your mat just might squeak.

Some practices, of course,
will start with distraction.
But practice with purpose,
and you'll find mindfulness in action.

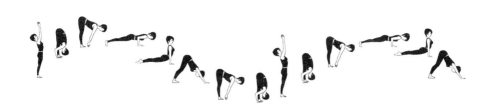

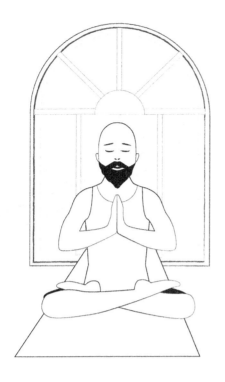

The process is the prize,
though a contest it's not.
It's the flexibility of your mind,
rather than tying into knots.
Look into yourself more,
and look out for yourself less.
You will finish your practice,
without being such a hot mess.

Use the pose as a tool,
to help shape your life off the mat.
An exercise for your soul,
and good vibes you'll attract.

So on the days that feel
you have nothing inside,
step onto your mat,
and just go along for the ride.

Make each movement matter,
and each matter glow.
The more that you practice,
the more you will grow!

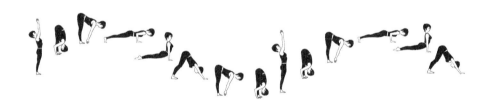

What you can't do, not important,
contrary to fact.

It's not where you can go,
but always going with tact!

And will you succeed?
Well, my friend, here's some news!
There's no #winning in yoga!
Trust your breath, you can't lose!

All you can do is your practice,
and soon you will see,
all will be coming,
99 percent guaranteed!

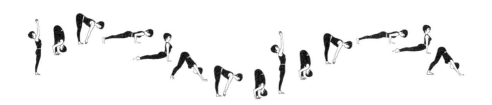

And oh, how you'll flow!
You will, the flow grows!

So…

Whether you are rigid or lanky,
can fit into a pocket.
Have joints that are double,
or creaky hip sockets.
Whether half the size of tall,
or the opposite of small,
you, too, can be a yogi,
especially if you fall.

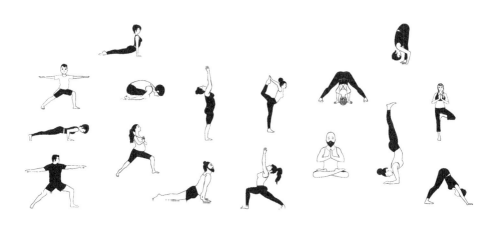

Just let go of your doubts.
Get out of your own way!

Child's Pose is waiting.
It's a new practice each day!

A Special Thanks

Endeavors like this always take a tribe.

To Carin Crook. Words can't appropriately describe my gratitude for all of the support and kindness you have shown me. Thank you for your friendship and your brilliant editing skills.

To Waylon Lewis and the staff at elephantjournal.com. For giving me the original platform to share my story.

To my mom. This book would not have happened without her full support and encouragement.

And to my dad. For unknowingly planting in me the seeds of a teacher. The apple does not fall far from the tree.

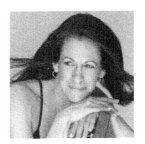

About The Author

Lyn Gerfin has been teaching yoga for more than 20 years. She owns a yoga studio in Ridgefield, Connecticut, where she also resides. Her articles have been featured online and in print.

For more information about her yoga, studio and other writings, visit lyngerfin.com.

Photo Credit: Kristen Jensen

CPSIA information can be obtained
at www.ICGtesting.com
Printed in the USA
BVOW09*1222260318

511596BV00005BA/39/P